CROSSFIT EXERCISE

For Beginners

A Comprehensive Guide To High-Intensity Workouts, Functional Fitness, And Building Strength And Endurance For A Healthier You

ROBERT LUGO

CHAPTER 1
Introduction To Crossfit

Introduction to CrossFit

CrossFit is a multifaceted fitness approach that combines elements of various disciplines such as weightlifting, gymnastics, and high-intensity interval training (HIIT). It focuses on functional movements performed at high intensity to improve overall fitness and performance across different domains. At its core, CrossFit aims to develop strength, endurance, flexibility, power, speed, coordination, agility, balance, and accuracy through diverse and challenging workouts.

What is CrossFit?

CrossFit can be defined as a strength and conditioning program that emphasizes constantly varied functional movements executed at high intensity.

It is designed to be scalable, making it suitable for individuals of all fitness levels, from beginners to elite athletes.

Workouts typically incorporate elements like weightlifting, bodyweight exercises, cardiovascular activities, and gymnastics movements, often performed in a time-constrained or competitive format.

History of CrossFit

The history of CrossFit traces back to the early 2000s when Greg Glassman and Lauren Jenai founded CrossFit, Inc. in Santa Cruz, California. Initially developed as a training method for police officers, firefighters, and military personnel, CrossFit gained popularity through its effectiveness in improving overall fitness and athletic performance.

Over the years, CrossFit has evolved into a global fitness phenomenon, with thousands of affiliated gyms (known as CrossFit boxes) worldwide and annual events like the CrossFit Games showcasing elite athletes' capabilities.

Benefits of CrossFit

CrossFit offers a range of benefits that appeal to fitness enthusiasts and athletes alike. One of its key advantages is its emphasis on functional movements, which are movements that mimic real-life activities and contribute to better overall performance in daily tasks and sports.

By incorporating a variety of exercises and workouts, CrossFit promotes physical adaptation and prevents plateauing, keeping workouts engaging and challenging. Additionally, the community aspect of CrossFit, with its supportive and competitive environment, fosters motivation, camaraderie, and accountability among participants.

CHAPTER 2
Getting Started With Crossfit

Getting Started with CrossFit involves several key aspects that are essential for beginners to understand. Firstly, finding a suitable CrossFit gym is crucial. These gyms are specifically designed for CrossFit workouts, which are known for their intensity and varied exercises.

When choosing a gym, factors such as location, facilities, coaching quality, and community atmosphere should be considered. Many CrossFit gyms offer introductory classes or sessions for beginners to familiarize themselves with the workouts and assess if CrossFit is suitable for their fitness goals.

Understanding CrossFit equipment is another vital aspect. CrossFit workouts often involve a range of equipment, including barbells, kettlebells, pull-up bars, rowing machines, and more. Each piece of equipment serves a specific purpose in CrossFit workouts, targeting different muscle groups and movement patterns. Beginners should learn how to use this equipment safely and effectively to maximize the benefits of their workouts while minimizing the risk of injury.

Safety precautions and warm-up techniques are fundamental in CrossFit. Due to the high-intensity nature of CrossFit workouts, proper warm-up routines are essential to prepare the body for exercise and reduce the risk of strains or injuries.

This includes dynamic stretches, mobility drills, and activation exercises that target key muscle groups used in CrossFit movements. Additionally, understanding and adhering to safety precautions, such as maintaining proper form, using appropriate weights, and knowing when to scale workouts, are crucial for a safe and effective CrossFit experience.

Overall, getting started with CrossFit requires finding a suitable gym, understanding the equipment used, and prioritizing safety through proper warm-up techniques and adherence to safety precautions. This foundational knowledge sets the stage for beginners to embark on their CrossFit journey with confidence and readiness to tackle challenging workouts effectively.

CHAPTER 3
Fundamental Crossfit Movements

Fundamental CrossFit Movements encompass a range of exercises that form the core of CrossFit training. These movements are foundational for building strength, power, and overall fitness.

One of the key movements in CrossFit is the squat. Squats target the lower body and are essential for developing leg strength. Air squats, which are bodyweight squats, are often used as a warm-up or endurance exercise. Front squats shift the emphasis to the quadriceps and core, challenging stability and strength. Overhead squats, where the weight is held above the head, require balance and flexibility, making them a comprehensive strength-building exercise.

Deadlifts are another fundamental movement in CrossFit. They primarily target the posterior chain, including the hamstrings, glutes, and lower back. Conventional deadlifts involve lifting the barbell from the floor with a shoulder-width stance, emphasizing hip hinge mechanics. Sumo deadlifts, with a wider stance and hands inside the knees, emphasize leg drive and hip extension.

Presses in CrossFit refer to overhead pressing movements that target the shoulders, triceps, and upper chest. The shoulder press is a basic movement where the weight is pressed overhead from shoulder height. Push press incorporates leg drive to generate momentum for heavier lifts, while push jerk involves a dynamic dip and drive to propel the weight overhead efficiently.

Pull-ups and their variations are crucial for upper body strength. Strict pull-ups emphasize controlled movement using primarily the back and arms. Kipping pull-ups add momentum from hip extension, allowing for faster repetitions. Butterfly pull-ups are a more advanced variation that involves a dynamic swinging motion for efficient cycling of reps.

Olympic lifts, including the clean jerk and snatch, are dynamic and explosive movements that require speed, power, and coordination. The clean and jerk involves lifting the barbell from the floor to the shoulders (clean) and then overhead (jerk) in a fluid motion. The snatch is a single movement where the barbell is lifted from the floor to overhead in one continuous motion, demanding precision and technique.

Gymnastics movements in CrossFit focus on bodyweight exercises that improve strength, coordination, and agility. Handstand push-ups target the shoulders and triceps while challenging balance and core stability. Muscle-ups combine a pull-up and a dip into one fluid movement, showcasing upper body strength and coordination. Toes-to-bar engages the core and hip flexors, requiring coordination and control to touch the toes to the pull-up bar.

Each of these fundamental CrossFit movements plays a crucial role in developing a well-rounded and functional fitness level.

They can be scaled and modified to suit individual fitness levels and goals, making them accessible to beginners while offering challenges to advanced athletes.

CHAPTER 4
Crossfit Workouts And Programming

CrossFit Workouts and Programming encompass a dynamic and multifaceted approach to fitness, blending elements of strength training, conditioning, and functional movements. Understanding WODs (Workout of the Day) is crucial in the CrossFit community, as it forms the backbone of daily training sessions.

These workouts are designed to be constantly varied, high intensity, and functional, aiming to improve overall fitness across ten recognized physical skills: cardiovascular/respiratory endurance, stamina, strength, flexibility, power, speed, coordination, agility, balance, and accuracy.

Designing Effective CrossFit Workouts involves a strategic combination of exercises that target different muscle groups and energy systems.

Variability is key, with workouts often incorporating elements such as weightlifting, gymnastics, and metabolic conditioning. Effective programming requires a balance between pushing boundaries to promote adaptation and avoiding overtraining or injury.

Scaling and Modifying Workouts for Different Levels is essential in CrossFit to accommodate varying fitness levels, abilities, and experience. Scaling involves adjusting workout parameters such as load, repetitions, and intensity to ensure that individuals can safely and effectively participate while still challenging themselves. Modifications may also be made based on specific goals, limitations, or progressions.

CrossFit Programming Principles guide the creation of balanced and effective training regimens. These principles include the use of functional movements that mimic real-life activities, performing workouts at high intensity to maximize results, focusing on compound movements for efficiency, constantly varying workouts to prevent plateaus and boredom, and incorporating rest and recovery to support overall fitness and performance gains.

By understanding these key concepts, CrossFit enthusiasts and trainers can create and participate in workouts that are both challenging and sustainable, leading to improved fitness, strength, and overall well-being.

CHAPTER 5

Nutrition And Recovery For Crossfit

Nutrition and Recovery play vital roles in optimizing performance and enhancing recovery for CrossFit athletes.

Nutrition is Important for CrossFit

Nutrition forms the foundation of athletic performance in CrossFit. Proper nutrition fuels workouts, supports muscle growth and repair and aids in recovery.

For CrossFit athletes, a balanced diet rich in macronutrients (carbohydrates, proteins, and fats) and micronutrients (vitamins and minerals) is crucial. Carbohydrates provide energy for high-intensity workouts, proteins support muscle repair and growth, and fats contribute to hormone production and overall health. Additionally, micronutrients play essential roles in various physiological processes, ensuring optimal performance and recovery.

Pre-Workout Nutrition

Pre-workout nutrition aims to fuel the body adequately for the upcoming training session. CrossFit athletes often benefit from consuming a combination of carbohydrates and proteins before workouts. Carbohydrates provide readily available energy, while proteins support muscle maintenance and readiness.

Foods such as bananas, whole grains, lean proteins, and smoothies with protein powder are popular choices for pre-workout meals. Timing is also crucial, with most athletes consuming a meal or snack containing carbohydrates and proteins approximately 1 to 2 hours before training.

Post-Workout Nutrition and Recovery Strategies

Post-workout nutrition is vital for replenishing glycogen stores, repairing muscle tissue, and promoting recovery. CrossFit athletes should prioritize consuming carbohydrates and proteins after training sessions to optimize these processes. Fast-digesting carbohydrates like fruits, rice, or potatoes help replenish glycogen, while proteins such as lean meats, fish, eggs, or protein shakes support muscle repair and growth. Including a source of healthy fats can also aid in nutrient absorption and overall recovery. Additionally, hydration plays a crucial role in recovery, with athletes needing to replenish fluids lost during exercise.

Hydration and Supplements for CrossFit Athletes

Proper hydration is essential for CrossFit athletes to maintain performance and prevent dehydration. Athletes should drink water throughout the day and during workouts to stay hydrated. Electrolytes, such as sodium, potassium, and magnesium, are also important for maintaining fluid balance and supporting muscle function. Sports drinks or electrolyte supplements can be beneficial, especially during intense or prolonged training sessions.

Supplements can complement a well-rounded diet for CrossFit athletes, but they should not replace whole foods. Common supplements used by CrossFit athletes include protein powders, creatine, branched-chain amino acids (BCAAs), and fish oil. These supplements can support muscle recovery, strength gains, and overall performance when used appropriately and in conjunction with a balanced diet.

nutrition and recovery strategies are integral components of success for CrossFit athletes.

By prioritizing proper nutrition, including pre-workout and post-workout meals, staying hydrated, and using supplements wisely, athletes can optimize their performance, support muscle recovery, and achieve their fitness goals effectively.

CHAPTER 6
Crossfit Competitions And Events

CrossFit competitions and events represent the pinnacle of athletic performance and endurance within the CrossFit community. These events encompass a range of challenges that test participants' strength, agility, endurance, and mental fortitude. Understanding the types of CrossFit competitions, preparing effectively for these events, and strategizing for success are critical aspects for any CrossFit athlete aiming to excel in competitive settings.

Types of CrossFit competitions vary widely, offering diverse challenges to athletes. The most common types include individual competitions, team competitions, and specialized events such as the CrossFit Games. Individual competitions pit athletes against each other in a series of workouts designed to push their limits across various domains, including weightlifting, gymnastics, and metabolic conditioning.

Team competitions, on the other hand, require coordination and synergy among team members to tackle collective challenges, often incorporating elements of communication and teamwork.

Specialized events like the CrossFit Games feature elite athletes competing in a series of grueling tests over several days, showcasing the pinnacle of CrossFit athleticism.

Preparing for a CrossFit competition demands a meticulous approach to training, recovery, and mental readiness. Athletes must focus on developing strength, endurance, and skill across a wide range of movements, including Olympic lifts, bodyweight exercises, and cardiovascular conditioning.

Structured training programs that emphasize periodization, skill development, and conditioning are essential to peak performance during competitions. Nutrition plays a crucial role in fueling training sessions and optimizing recovery, with a focus on macronutrient balance, hydration, and supplementation to support athletic demands.

Strategies for success in CrossFit competitions extend beyond physical preparation to mental resilience and strategic planning.

Athletes must cultivate a positive mindset, resilience to adversity, and adaptability to unpredictable challenges that may arise during competition.

Mental skills training, visualization techniques, and mindfulness practices can enhance focus, confidence, and performance under pressure. Strategic planning involves understanding competition formats, pacing strategies, and maximizing strengths while mitigating weaknesses to achieve optimal results.

CrossFit competitions and events represent a unique and demanding platform for showcasing athletic prowess and competitive spirit within the CrossFit community.

By understanding the types of competitions, preparing effectively through structured training and nutrition, and implementing strategies for success encompassing both physical and mental aspects, athletes can elevate their performance and achieve success in the dynamic and challenging world of CrossFit competition.

CHAPTER 7
Crossfit For Special Populations

CrossFit, with its emphasis on functional movements performed at high intensity, can be tailored to suit various populations, including beginners, women, older adults, and athletes with disabilities. Each of these groups brings unique considerations and challenges, requiring specialized approaches within the CrossFit framework.

CrossFit for Beginners:

For newcomers to CrossFit, a gradual introduction to the program is essential to prevent injuries and build foundational strength and skill. Beginners often start with learning proper movement mechanics, focusing on bodyweight exercises before progressing to more complex movements and heavier loads. Emphasis is placed on technique and safety, with workouts tailored to individual fitness levels.

CrossFit for beginners also involves education on nutrition, recovery, and the CrossFit methodology to ensure a holistic approach to fitness.

CrossFit for Women:

CrossFit has gained popularity among women for its empowering and inclusive environment. Workouts for women in CrossFit often incorporate a mix of strength training, cardio, and functional movements to improve overall fitness and athleticism. Special attention is given to exercises that target areas of strength commonly associated with women's fitness goals, such as lower body strength, core stability, and functional endurance. CrossFit for Women also emphasizes community support, camaraderie, and body positivity.

CrossFit for Older Adults:

CrossFit is increasingly recognized as a beneficial fitness program for older adults, offering tailored workouts that focus on mobility, balance, strength, and cardiovascular health.

Programs for older adults in CrossFit often include modified movements, lower intensity options, and longer warm-up and cool-down periods to accommodate age-related changes in fitness and mobility. CrossFit for older adults aims to improve quality of life, functional independence, and overall well-being through safe and effective exercise programming.

CrossFit for Athletes with Disabilities:

CrossFit's adaptable nature makes it accessible to athletes with disabilities, offering modified workouts and equipment adaptations to accommodate different abilities and mobility levels. CrossFit for athletes with disabilities focuses on inclusive training environments, personalized coaching, and creative exercise modifications to optimize performance and promote fitness goals. Emphasis is placed on functional movements, skill development, and adaptive strategies to overcome challenges and achieve success in CrossFit training.

Each of these specialized populations within CrossFit highlights the program's versatility and inclusivity, catering to diverse fitness needs and goals. Through tailored programming, education, and support, CrossFit continues to empower individuals of all backgrounds to pursue fitness, health, and performance excellence.

CHAPTER 8
Crossfit Community And Culture

Building a Supportive CrossFit Community

Building a supportive CrossFit community is not merely about bringing individuals together for workouts; it encompasses a deeper ethos of camaraderie, mutual encouragement, and shared goals. Central to this ethos is the concept of the "box," the term used to describe a CrossFit gym. Within the box, members forge connections that extend beyond physical fitness, creating a sense of belonging and accountability.

At the heart of a supportive CrossFit community are the coaches. These individuals play a pivotal role in fostering a positive environment by providing guidance, motivation, and personalized attention to each member. Coaches in CrossFit often embody the principles they teach, serving as role models for dedication, perseverance, and teamwork.

One of the key factors in building a strong community is effective communication. CrossFit boxes often utilize various communication channels, such as social media groups, newsletters, and community events, to keep members informed and engaged.

Regular updates on workouts, nutrition tips, and success stories contribute to a sense of shared progress and achievement.

In addition to formal communication channels, informal interactions within the box contribute significantly to community building.

The camaraderie that develops during workouts, the friendly competition during WODs (Workout of the Day), and the post-workout conversations all contribute to a supportive and inclusive atmosphere.

Moreover, a supportive CrossFit community extends beyond the walls of the box. Many CrossFit enthusiasts participate in community outreach programs, charity events, and fitness challenges that not only promote physical well-being but also contribute to social causes and community development. These initiatives strengthen bonds among members and showcase the positive impact of CrossFit beyond individual fitness goals.

Ethical and Safety Considerations in CrossFit

Ethical and safety considerations are paramount in CrossFit, given its high-intensity nature and diverse participant demographics.

CrossFit coaches and trainers undergo rigorous training and certification processes to ensure they are equipped to provide safe and effective workouts for all levels of fitness.

One of the fundamental ethical considerations in CrossFit is maintaining a focus on individual progress and health over competition. While friendly competition can be motivating, it is essential to prioritize proper form, technique, and injury prevention.

Coaches play a crucial role in enforcing these principles and guiding members toward sustainable fitness practices.

Safety protocols are integral to every CrossFit box, encompassing equipment maintenance, facility cleanliness, and emergency preparedness.

Coaches undergo training in CPR, first aid, and injury prevention to handle unforeseen situations effectively. Additionally, CrossFit boxes often collaborate with healthcare professionals to provide comprehensive support to members with specific health concerns or injuries.

Another ethical aspect of CrossFit is inclusivity and diversity. CrossFit embraces individuals of all ages, fitness levels, and backgrounds, fostering an environment where everyone feels welcomed and supported. Coaches are trained to adapt workouts and scales for diverse needs, ensuring that every member can participate safely and achieve their fitness goals.

CrossFit also emphasizes ethical conduct in competitions and events, promoting fair play, sportsmanship, and respect for fellow athletes. The community ethos extends to competitions, where participants cheer for each other, celebrate achievements, and embody the spirit of sportsmanship.

The Role of CrossFit in Fitness Culture

CrossFit has emerged as a significant influencer in fitness culture, shaping trends, attitudes, and approaches to physical wellness. At its core, CrossFit challenges conventional fitness norms by promoting functional movements, varied workouts, and measurable results. This approach has resonated with a wide range of individuals seeking dynamic and effective fitness solutions.

One of the key contributions of CrossFit to fitness culture is its emphasis on functional fitness.

Unlike traditional gym workouts that may focus on isolated muscle groups, CrossFit workouts incorporate movements that mimic real-life activities, improving overall strength, agility, and flexibility. This functional approach has gained traction not only among athletes but also among everyday fitness enthusiasts looking to enhance their daily activities.

CrossFit's emphasis on intensity and variability has also influenced workout programming across the fitness industry. Concepts like HIIT (High-Intensity Interval Training) and circuit training draw inspiration from CrossFit's structured yet adaptable approach to workouts. This has led to a broader recognition of the benefits of diverse training modalities in achieving comprehensive fitness goals.

Moreover, CrossFit's community-centric model has redefined the social aspect of fitness. By fostering supportive communities within and beyond the gym, CrossFit has created a sense of belonging and motivation that extends beyond individual workouts. This community-driven approach has inspired other fitness communities to prioritize inclusivity, support, and collective progress.

CrossFit's impact on fitness culture goes beyond physical training; it encompasses values of community, ethics, and holistic well-being. By building supportive communities, emphasizing safety and ethics, and redefining fitness norms, CrossFit continues to shape the landscape of modern fitness culture.

CHAPTER 9
Crossfit And Mental Health

CrossFit, beyond its physical benefits, has gained recognition for its positive impact on mental health. The Psychological Benefits of CrossFit encompass a range of aspects that contribute to overall well-being.

Firstly, CrossFit fosters a sense of community and belonging among participants. The group dynamics, camaraderie, and shared goals create a supportive environment that can enhance mental resilience and reduce feelings of isolation or loneliness.

Additionally, the structured nature of CrossFit workouts, often incorporating varied movements and challenges, can stimulate cognitive functions and improve mental agility.

Using CrossFit as a Stress Reliever is a common strategy adopted by many individuals seeking to manage stress effectively.

The intense physical activity involved in CrossFit workouts triggers the release of endorphins, which are natural mood lifters and stress reducers.

The focus required during workouts also serves as a distraction from daily stressors, allowing participants to channel their energy into productive physical exertion. Moreover, the goal-oriented nature of CrossFit, with measurable progress in fitness levels, provides a sense of achievement and empowerment, further aiding in stress management.

Addressing Mental Health Challenges in CrossFit involves understanding and accommodating diverse needs within the community.

CrossFit gyms and coaches play a crucial role in creating inclusive environments where mental health concerns are acknowledged and supported. This may involve offering modified workouts for individuals dealing with anxiety or depression, providing resources for mental health education, and encouraging open communication about mental well-being.

By promoting a holistic approach to health that includes both physical and mental aspects, CrossFit can contribute positively to overall mental wellness.

CHAPTER 10
Advanced Crossfit Techniques

Advanced CrossFit Techniques encompass a realm of specialized skills and training methodologies that push the boundaries of traditional fitness routines. This section delves into three key areas: Advanced Strength Training Methods, Advanced Gymnastics Skills, and Advanced Olympic Lifting Techniques, each of which plays a crucial role in enhancing performance and achieving peak athletic abilities in CrossFit.

Advanced Strength Training Methods in CrossFit go beyond basic weightlifting principles. They incorporate advanced techniques such as cluster sets, wave loading, and eccentric training to maximize muscle hypertrophy and strength gains. Cluster sets involve breaking up a set into smaller clusters with short rest intervals, allowing for higher intensity and volume. Wave loading alternates between heavy and moderate loads within a set to challenge muscles differently and stimulate greater adaptation.

 Eccentric training focuses on the lowering phase of an exercise, emphasizing controlled muscle lengthening for increased muscle damage and growth.

Moving on to Advanced Gymnastics Skills, CrossFit athletes aspire to master movements like muscle-ups, handstand walks, and advanced bar work. These skills require exceptional body control, core strength, and coordination. Progressions in gymnastics training involve mastering basic movements like pull-ups and push-ups before advancing to more complex exercises such as kipping pull-ups and handstand push-ups. Advanced gymnastics drills emphasize technique refinement, spatial awareness, and dynamic transitions between movements, contributing to fluidity and efficiency in workouts.

In the realm of Advanced Olympic Lifting Techniques, CrossFit blends elements of weightlifting with functional fitness to optimize power and speed. Athletes focus on lifts like the snatch, clean, and jerk, aiming for precision, speed, and explosive power. Advanced techniques include complex variations like squat snatches, split jerks, and hang cleans, challenging athletes to coordinate multiple joint movements seamlessly. Olympic lifting drills emphasize timing, speed under the bar, and efficient force generation, vital for success in CrossFit competitions and challenging workouts.

CrossFit's emphasis on advanced techniques underscores its commitment to continuous improvement and athletic excellence. By mastering Advanced Strength Training Methods, Advanced Gymnastics Skills, and Advanced Olympic Lifting Techniques, athletes elevate their performance levels, conquer new fitness milestones, and thrive in the dynamic, demanding world of CrossFit.

CHAPTER 11
Crossfit Coaching And Leadership

Qualities of a Good CrossFit Coach

A good CrossFit coach embodies a unique set of qualities that go beyond mere knowledge of exercises and techniques. To begin with, having strong communication skills is essential.Coaches must be able to articulate instructions clearly, motivate athletes, and provide constructive feedback. Patience is another key attribute, as CrossFit workouts can be challenging, requiring coaches to remain calm and supportive even in intense situations. Adaptability is crucial, as coaches need to tailor workouts to individual needs while maintaining the overall program's integrity. Empathy plays a vital role in understanding athletes' struggles and fostering a positive training environment.

Furthermore, a good coach exhibits leadership by example, demonstrating proper form, dedication, and a strong work ethic.

They are knowledgeable about injury prevention and safety protocols, ensuring that athletes train safely and effectively. Professionalism is non-negotiable, encompassing punctuality, organization, and respect for athletes' privacy and boundaries. A good coach is also a lifelong learner, staying updated on industry trends, attending workshops, and seeking continuous improvement. Ultimately, the best coaches inspire and empower their athletes to achieve their full potential, both physically and mentally.

Techniques for Coaching CrossFit

Coaching techniques in CrossFit blend scientific knowledge with practical application to optimize athlete performance. Coaches utilize effective cueing, using concise and specific instructions to guide athletes through movements. Visual demonstrations are valuable, allowing athletes to see proper form and technique in action.

Feedback loops, such as video analysis and immediate corrections, enhance learning and skill development. Coaches also employ progressive overload, gradually increasing intensity and complexity to challenge athletes while avoiding injury.

Periodization is a key coaching strategy, structuring training cycles to balance workload, recovery, and performance peaks. Variability is essential, incorporating diverse workouts to prevent plateaus and maintain motivation. Coaches integrate goal setting, helping athletes define clear objectives and track progress over time.

Individualization is paramount, adjusting workouts based on athletes' abilities, limitations, and goals. Coaches also foster a supportive team environment, encouraging camaraderie, sportsmanship, and mutual support among athletes.

Building Leadership Skills in CrossFit

Building leadership skills in CrossFit involves cultivating qualities like vision, communication, collaboration, and mentorship. Leaders set a compelling vision for the team, aligning goals with values and inspiring others to strive for excellence. Effective communication is essential, fostering open dialogue, active listening, and clarity of expectations. Collaboration is encouraged, promoting teamwork, shared decision-making, and leveraging collective strengths.

Mentorship plays a crucial role in leadership development, with experienced athletes mentoring newcomers and coaches guiding athletes' growth. Leaders prioritize personal development, continuously learning, adapting, and seeking feedback to improve themselves and their teams. They lead by example, demonstrating integrity, resilience, and a commitment to continuous improvement.

Empowering others is central to leadership in CrossFit, encouraging autonomy, creativity, and accountability among team members.

Building leadership skills in CrossFit requires a holistic approach that combines vision, communication, collaboration, mentorship, and personal development. Effective leaders inspire, empower, and unite their teams, fostering a culture of excellence, growth, and camaraderie.

CHAPTER 12
crossfit and injury prevention

CrossFit, known for its intensity and varied workouts, is not without its risks, particularly regarding injuries. Understanding common CrossFit injuries and strategies for prevention is crucial for athletes and trainers alike to ensure a safe training environment and promote long-term fitness success.

Common CrossFit injuries encompass a range of issues, from overuse injuries like tendonitis and stress fractures to acute injuries such as muscle strains and joint dislocations. These injuries often stem from improper technique, overtraining, or inadequate recovery. For instance, improper form during weightlifting movements like deadlifts or squats can lead to back injuries, while excessive high-impact exercises without sufficient rest can contribute to stress fractures or tendon injuries.

To avoid these injuries, athletes must prioritize proper form and technique over speed or intensity. This includes mastering fundamental movements before progressing to more complex exercises and using appropriate weights for individual fitness levels. Additionally, incorporating rest days into training schedules and varying workouts to prevent overuse of specific muscle groups can mitigate injury risks.

Recovery strategies play a vital role in managing CrossFit-related injuries. Active recovery, such as light stretching, yoga, or low-intensity cardio, can promote blood flow and aid in muscle recovery without exacerbating existing injuries. Physical therapy and targeted rehabilitation exercises can also help athletes recover from injuries and prevent recurrence.

Creating a safe training environment in CrossFit gyms involves several key practices. Trainers should prioritize proper warm-ups and cooldowns to prepare muscles for exercise and prevent abrupt transitions that can strain muscles or joints. Equipment maintenance and regular safety checks are essential to identify potential hazards like worn-out gear or slippery floors.

Educating athletes about injury prevention techniques and the importance of listening to their bodies' signals is fundamental to creating a culture of safety within CrossFit communities. Encouraging open communication between athletes and trainers regarding any discomfort or pain during workouts can prompt timely interventions and prevent injuries from worsening.

Mitigating CrossFit-related injuries requires a multifaceted approach that emphasizes proper technique, adequate recovery strategies, and a safe training environment. By implementing these strategies, athletes can enjoy the benefits of CrossFit training while minimizing the risk of injuries that can hinder their progress and overall fitness journey.

CHAPTER 13
Crossfit For Long-Term Fitness

CrossFit is not just a short-term fitness trend but a lifestyle approach that can be integrated into long-term fitness plans. Incorporating CrossFit into a long-term fitness plan involves understanding its principles and how they align with sustained health and wellness goals. This integration requires a thoughtful approach to training, progression, and adaptation over time.

Periodization and progression are crucial aspects of CrossFit training for long-term fitness success. Periodization involves organizing training into specific blocks or cycles, each with its own focus and intensity level. This structured approach allows for systematic progression while preventing burnout and overtraining. In CrossFit, periodization can be applied to various aspects such as strength training, metabolic conditioning, and skill development.

CrossFit for aging athletes presents unique considerations and opportunities. As individuals age, their fitness needs and capabilities evolve. CrossFit offers a versatile framework that can be tailored to accommodate age-related changes while promoting functional fitness and overall well-being. Strategies for older athletes may include modifications to workouts, emphasis on mobility and flexibility, and targeted programming to address specific age-related challenges.

Incorporating CrossFit into a long-term fitness plan requires strategic planning, periodization, and consideration of individual needs and goals. By understanding the principles of CrossFit and adapting them to suit long-term fitness objectives, individuals can enjoy the benefits of this dynamic training approach throughout their fitness journey.

Conclusion

In the dynamic world of CrossFit, your journey doesn't end with mastering a few moves or hitting a personal best.

It's a continuous evolution, a lifestyle that transforms not just your body but your mindset and resilience. As you conclude this comprehensive guide, you've delved into the depths of CrossFit, from its humble origins to its profound impact on fitness culture and mental well-being.

You've learned the fundamental movements that form the backbone of CrossFit, from squats to Olympic lifts, embracing the challenge of pushing your limits and discovering new strengths. You've explored the art of designing effective workouts and programming, understanding that CrossFit is not just about intensity but also about intelligent progression and adaptation.

Nutrition and recovery have become pillars of your CrossFit journey, understanding that fueling your body right and prioritizing recovery are non-negotiable for peak performance.

You've glimpsed into the world of CrossFit competitions, where grit meets strategy, and success is defined by determination and preparation.

CrossFit isn't just for the elite; it's for everyone. You've discovered how it caters to special populations, empowering beginners, women, older adults, and athletes with disabilities to embrace their potential and thrive.

You've witnessed the power of community, where support and camaraderie fuel your progress, and safety and ethics ensure a sustainable fitness culture.

Your journey doesn't end here; it's a lifelong commitment to health, growth, and self-discovery. As you embrace advanced techniques, coaching, injury prevention, and long-term fitness strategies, remember that CrossFit isn't just about what you can do today; it's about building a better tomorrow, one workout at a time. So keep pushing, keep learning, and keep evolving.